No Carb Cookbook for A Successful and Easy Weight Loss

The Most Delicious No Carb Meals in One Cookbook

Table of Contents

Introduction

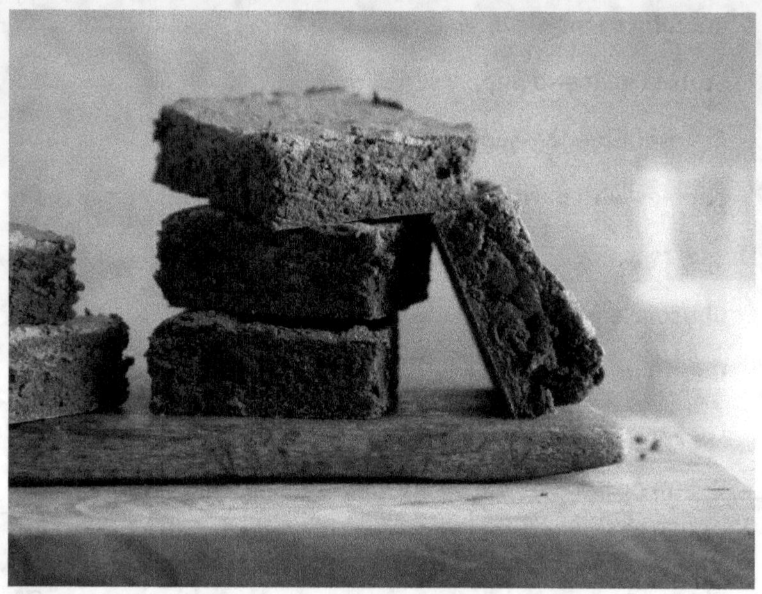

Ready to embrace the new way of losing weight? Carbohydrates are the ones to blame. A diet that doesn't include any of them will work for you. At this moment, you might ask yourself: Is this really possible? How do I cook some no-carb meals? Will I spend more money on buying food? Will the process of searching for recipes and cooking take lots of time?

You really don't have to worry about anything. We have everything sorted out for you. The No carb cookbook has a carefully picked selection of delicious meals that will melt down the calories for you. The best thing is that the recipes don't contain any fancy ingredients that require you to go to specialized shops. They work with very basic ingredients that you already have in your kitchen. All you have to do is follow the simple instructions. You won't lose your precious time searching to see if the ingredients are suitable or not.

Don't miss your chance to make a positive life change today. We invite you to take a look at these easy no carb recipes!

Appetizers

Zero carb bread recipe

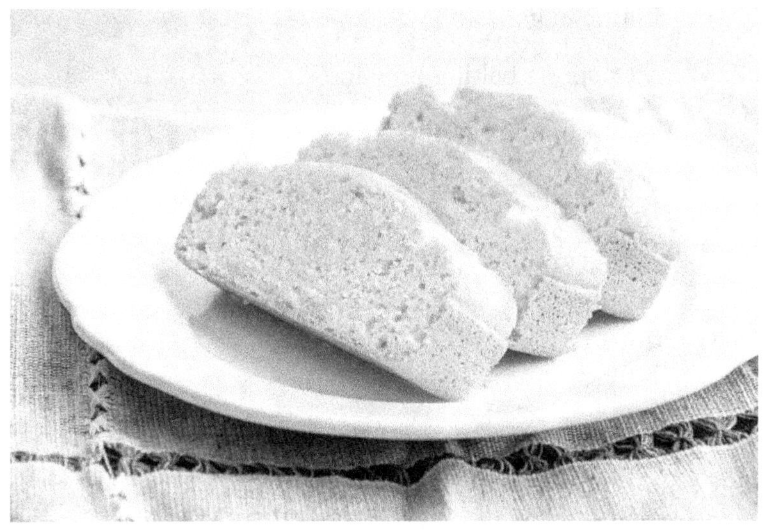

Bread is one of those guilty pleasures that keep us away from weight loss. But, this recipe will change your life. The zero carb bread recipe is so delicious and will satisfy those cravings. The best thing is that, as the name says, it doesn't have any carbs. You are free to enjoy this easy to make bread. So, let's get started!

Servings:10

Cooking time: 30 minutes

Ingredients

- 3 large eggs
- ¼ teaspoon baking powder
- 3 Tablespoons cream cheese
- Salt
- garlic powder

Instructions

1. Start by separating the whites from the yolks. Add the yolks into a bowl.

2. Add the cream cheese in the bowl with the yolks. Mix until smooth/.

3. Add the whites into a second bowl. Add in baking powder. Beat with a hand mixer on high speed. You are finished when it is fluffy and stiff peaks form.

4. Add the mixture with the egg yolks to the second bowl. Do this slowly and carefully, so that you won't break the fluffiness. Mix.

5. Using a spoon, add 10 to 12 even circles on baking paper. Sprinkle with garlic powder.

6. Bake for 17 to 20 minutes on 300 degrees, or until golden brown.

Easy pepperoni chips

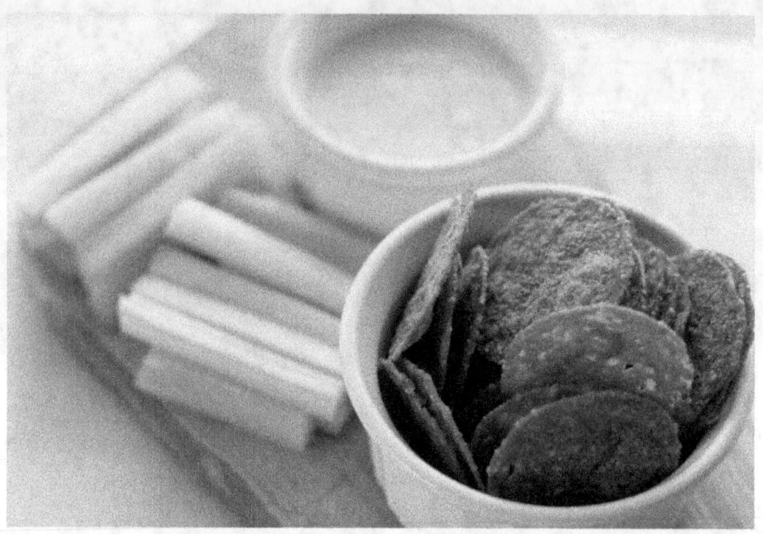

Are you craving for some crispy and crunchy snacks? Don't worry, because there are so many delicious snacks that are entirely carb-free. These pepperoni chips are one easy and tasty recipe that anyone can prepare. The process will only take you five minutes, so head to the kitchen right now!

Servings:2

Cooking time: 15 minutes

Ingredients

- 4 oz pepperoni

Instructions

1. Start by turning the oven to broil.

2. Line a sheet with baking paper. Place the pepperoni slices in one layer. Make sure that they don't cover each other.

3. Bake for 1.5- to 2 minutes, or until brown on the edges.

4. Transfer to a plate and let them cool for 10 minutes, or until the chips harden.

Aromatic cheese breadsticks

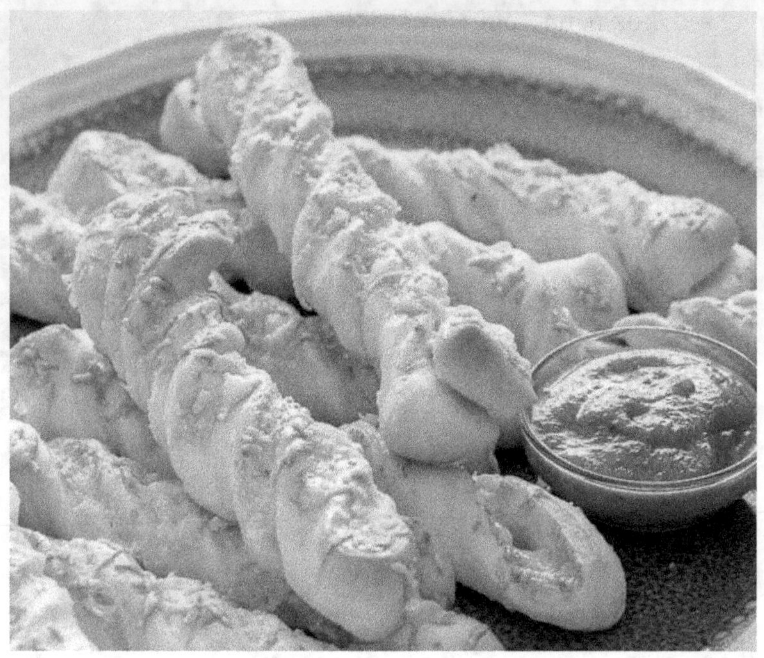

Craving for a rich snack or appetizer? These cheese breadsticks are the perfect recipe. You can make them in so little time. Munch during movie night, or pack them for work. They are an excellent combination of cheese so that they will keep you full in between meals. Plus, you can make them as an appetizer for your guests. The possibilities are endless, so let's get started!

Servings:2

Cooking time: 25 minutes

Ingredients

- 1 cup grated parmesan cheese
- 1 cup shredded mozzarella
- 1 large egg
- 1 teaspoon garlic powder

Instructions

1. Preheat oven to 350.

2. Put the cheese, egg, and garlic in a bowl. Mix well until combined.

3. Line a baking sheet with paper. Place the mixture. Flatten it out until you reach a thin dough.

4. Bake for 15 minutes. Then, broil for a few minutes so that the top will get golden brown color.

Coconut flour biscuits in a mug

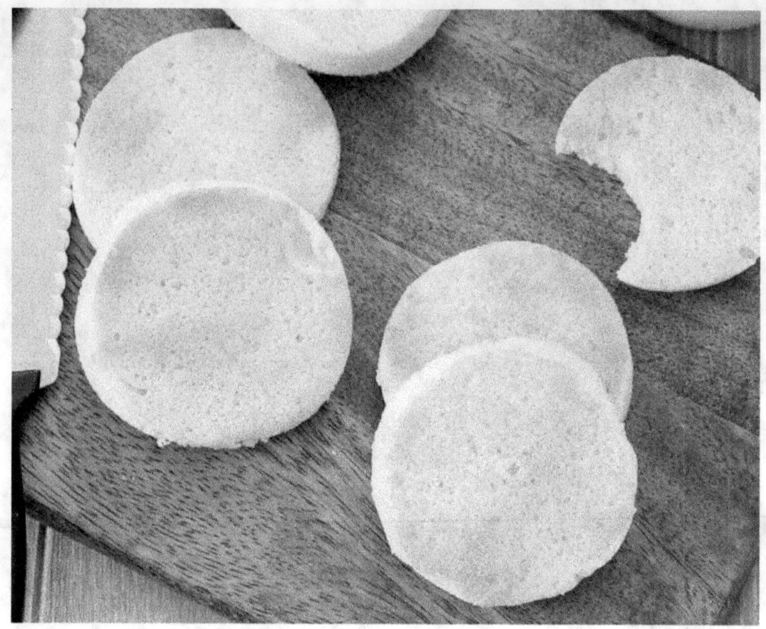

Are you craving for crunchy biscuits that you can dip in your no-carb dippings? Get ready for the 5-minute recipe that will amaze everyone. The best part is that this recipe will be made in the microwave, in only one bow. These easy coconut flour biscuits are a great snack or an appetizer. Even beginners will be able to cook it, so let's move to the **Instructions**!

Servings: 1

Cooking time: 5 minutes

Ingredients

- 2 tablespoons Coconut flour
- 1 tablespoon butter
- 1 tablespoon Heavy Whipping Cream
- 1 Egg
- 1/4 teaspoon Baking powder
- 1/4 cup Cheddar Cheese
- 2 tablespoons Water
- 1/8 teaspoon Dried Parsley
- 1/8 teaspoon garlic powder
- 1/8 teaspoon Onion powder
- 1/8 teaspoon salt
- 1/8 teaspoon freshly ground pepper

Instructions

1. Start by melting the butter. You can do this easily by microwaving it in a microwave-safe mug for 20 seconds.

2. Add in flour, baking powder, and the spices. Mix well with a fork.

3. Next, add the egg, water, cheese, and heavy whipping cream in the mug. Mix well again.

4. Get it back in the micro and set the timer to 3 minutes. Remove from the mug carefully and leave it to cool before you slice.

Salad in bacon basket finger food

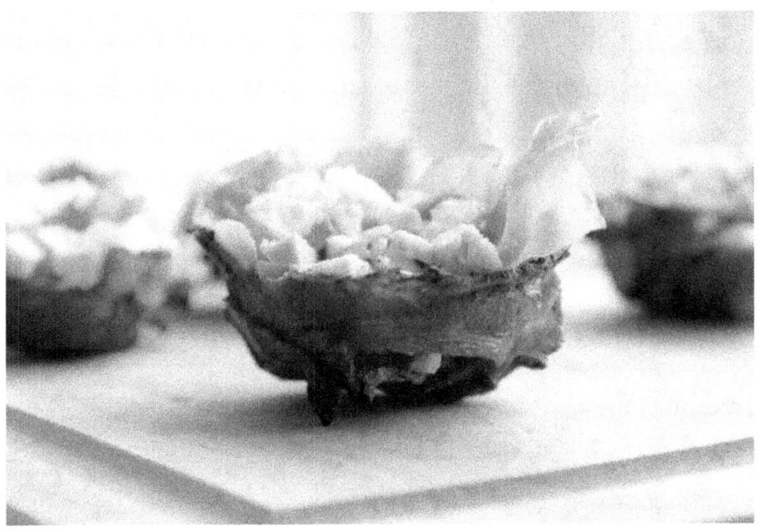

Whether you want a gourmet appetizer, a transportable lunch that you can pack for work, or something to serve to your guests, this is the recipe to hold onto. The crispy and crunchy baskets are filled with fresh and aromatic Caesar salad. Quick, simple, but incredibly delicious. No one will ever suppose that this finger food will contribute to weight loss. So, let's get started!

Servings:4

Cooking time:60 minutes

Ingredients

- 8 slices bacon
- ½ cup diced slicing tomato
- ½ cup lettuce
- 2 ounces grated Parmesan cheese
- 1/3 cup Caesar salad dressing
- Salt and pepper to taste

Instructions

1. Preheat oven to 400 degrees.

2. Cut each slice of bacon in half.

3. Take a muffin tin. Turn it upside down. To make the baskets, cross two slices over the pockets. Then, wrap two slices around the sides. You should have 2 in total.

4. Place the upside-down muffin tin on a baking sheet and bake for 20 minutes. Remove the baskets with a fork and return to the oven for 5-10 minutes. Remove and let them cool for 15 minutes.

5. Chop the lettuce to small pieces.

6. Mix with tomato and top with dressing. Place the salad into the baskets.

7. Top with some parmesan and enjoy!

Bacon Pinwheels with Cream Cheese

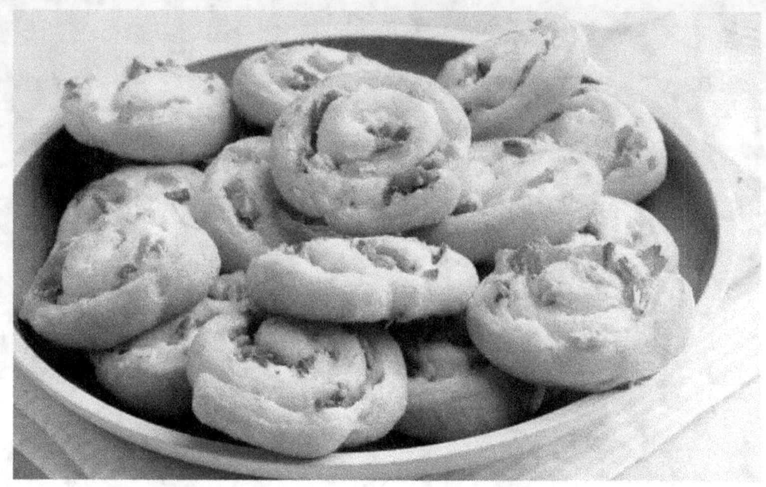

Pinwheels are one easy and delicious appetizer or snack. But, did you know that you can prepare a no-carb version? This recipe will give you complete information on how to do it. Layer your **Ingredients**, roll it, slice it, and you have the perfect lunch for work. You can pack each piece individually in plastic wrap so that you have your snack ready to go. Let's get started with the recipe!

Servings: 10

Cooking time: 15 minutes

Ingredients

- 7 slices cooked bacon
- 8 slices thick-sliced ham
- 1/4 cup chopped olives
- 4 oz cream cheese, softened
- 1-1/2 teaspoons ranch seasoning

Instructions

1. Layer the ham on a cutting board. Overlap rows 4x2.

2. Add the softened cream cheese. Spread it evenly with a knife on the ham.

3. Drizzle with ranch seasoning for taste. Sprinkle with chopped olives.

4. Lay the bacon on top.

5. Tightly roll the ham. Cut with a sharp knife to 1-2 inch pieces. Enjoy!

Delicious turkey meat wrap

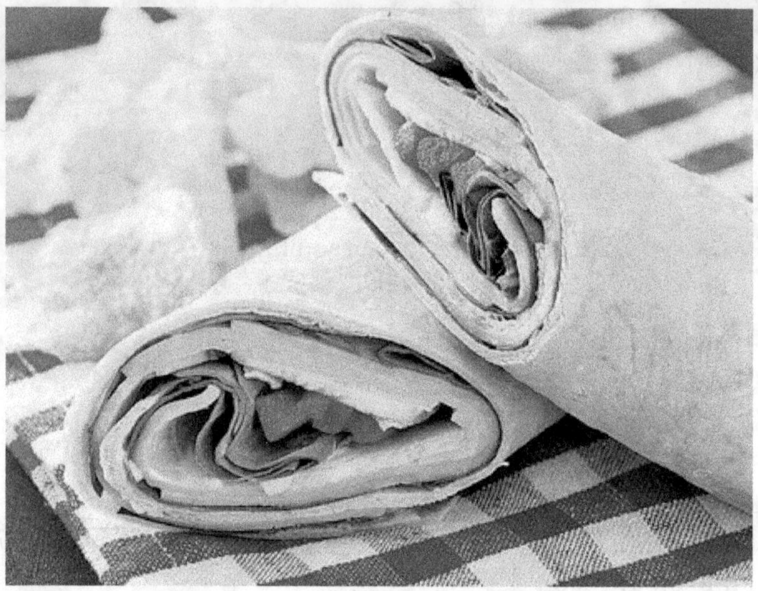

Do you love the taste of good old wrap? You must enjoy all those flavors and fillings, layer by layer. When eating no carb, you think that you won't enjoy your favorite meal anymore. But, this time you will be so happy to find out that it works for no-carb too. This recipe will give you clear **Instructions** on how to prepare the perfect wrap. It uses turkey meat instead of a tortilla that is full of carbs. The taste is guaranteed to be perfect, so let's get started!

Servings: 1

Cooking time: 5 minutes

Ingredients

- 4 oz cream cheese, softened
- 1 medium-thick slice deli turkey
- 1-2 strips of cucumber
- 2-4 strips of red bell peppers

Instructions

1. On a cutting board, layer the turkey slices.

2. Spread with cream cheese evenly on top.

3. Then, layer the strips of bell pepper. Continue with the cucumber. The vegetables will bring a dose of freshness to the meal.

4. Roll it up carefully. Slice the wraps with a sharp knife. Now, you are free to enjoy them!

Crunchy vinegar zucchini chips

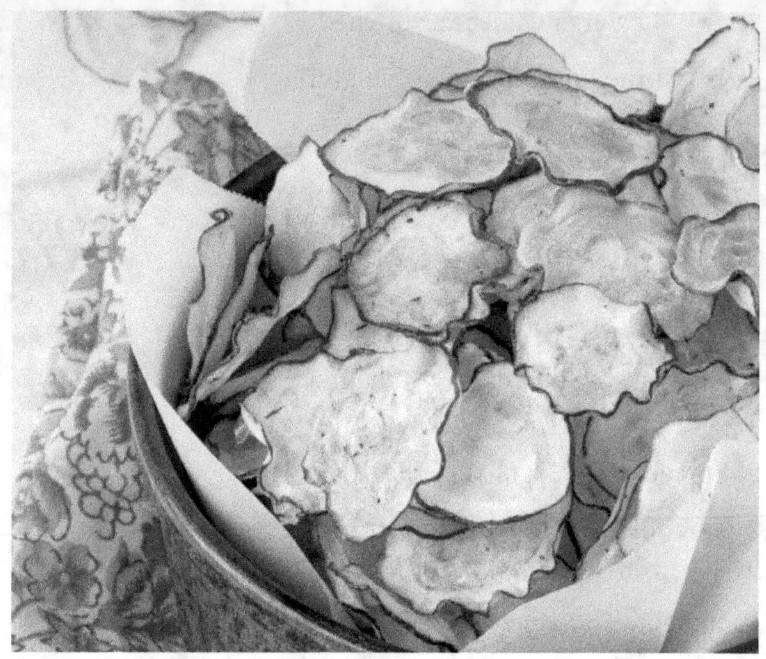

Here is another extremely delicious recipe for a snack that won't add up on the calories. These zucchini chips are the perfect replacement for the usual potato chips. You will be amazed by the crunchy, salty, and tasty snack. Whether you eat it on a movie night with friends, or just share with your family, the pleasure is guaranteed. So, let's get to the recipe!

Servings: 8

Cooking time: 3 hours

Ingredients

- 4 cups thinly sliced zucchini
- 2 tablespoons white balsamic vinegar
- 2 teaspoons salt
- 2 tablespoons olive oil

Instructions

1. Prepare the dressing first. Mix together the olive oil and vinegar.

2. Place the thin zucchini slices in a bowl. Pour with the dressing and toss.

3. Line a baking sheet with paper. Lay the slices so that they don't cover each other.

4. Preheat to 200 degrees and bake for 2-3 hours. Remember to turn them, so that they will cook evenly. Enjoy!

Breakfast

Spongy no-carb pancakes

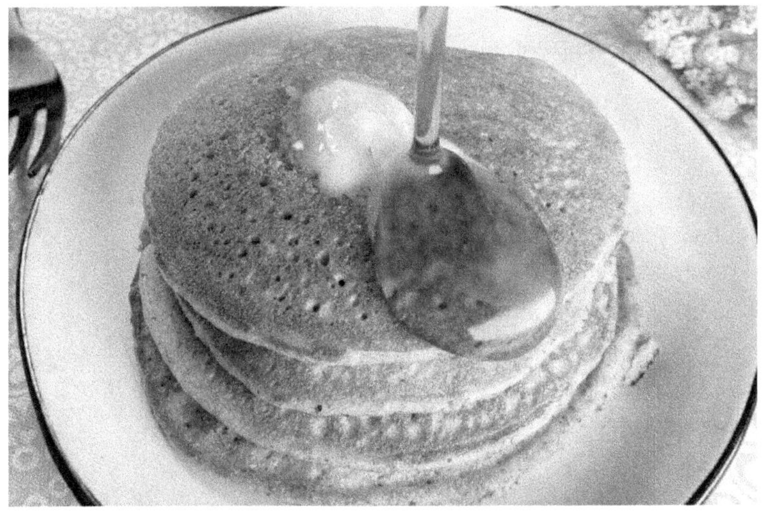

Are you craving for fluffy and delicious pancakes? Don't worry, because this recipe is here to prove you that tasty can be no carb too. This recipe will give you complete **Instructions** on how to prepare the best pancakes ever. They are so spongy, moist, and fluffy, so you won't even notice that they are carb-free.

Servings:4

Cooking time: 14 minutes

Ingredients

- 1/4 cup coconut flour

- 1 cup almond flour
- 1 teaspoon salt
- 2 tablespoons of low-calorie natural sweetener
- 6 large eggs
- 1 teaspoon baking powder
- 1 teaspoon pure vanilla extract
- 1/4 cup of heavy whipping cream
- 2 tablespoons of butter, melted

Instructions

1. Mix the dry **Ingredients**: almond flour, coconut flour, baking powder, sweetener, and salt.

2. Make sure that eggs and heavy cream are at room temperature. Whisk them into the dry **Ingredients**, together with butter and vanilla.

3. Heat an oiled pan over medium-high.

4. Add batter. Cook until you see bubbles. The edges should be cooked too. 3 to 4 minutes is enough on each side.

5. Repeat until you are out of batter. Enjoy!

Savory breakfast bowl

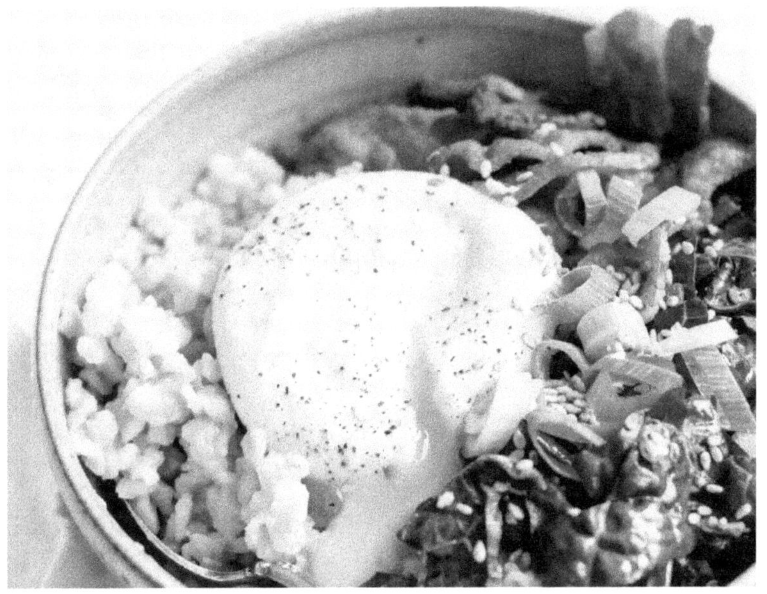

Do you love to have savory things for breakfast? This recipe is meant to keep you full until lunch. With having no carbs, it is the perfect choice for the people that want to lose weight and avoid feeling hungry. It is a quick and easy one, and everyone can do it. The most important trick behind this recipe is the right balance of **Ingredients**. So, let;s get started!

Servings: 1

Cooking time: 5 minutes

Ingredients

- 3 slices bacon, sliced
- 2 eggs
- 3 cups collard greens
- 1/2 teaspoon salt
- 1/4 teaspoon freshly ground pepper
- 1/4 teaspoon garlic powder
- 1/2 tablespoon butter

Instructions

Grab a skillet. Heat it to medium-high. Add pieces of bacon and cook.

Add in the greens. Sprinkle garlic powder, salt, and pepper. Cook until softened. Add them into a bowl.

Add the butter into the pan. Add in the cracked eggs and let them fry. Season with salt and pepper to taste. Once the white is cooked, transform them into the bowl. Enjoy your breakfast!

Eggs in avocado recipe

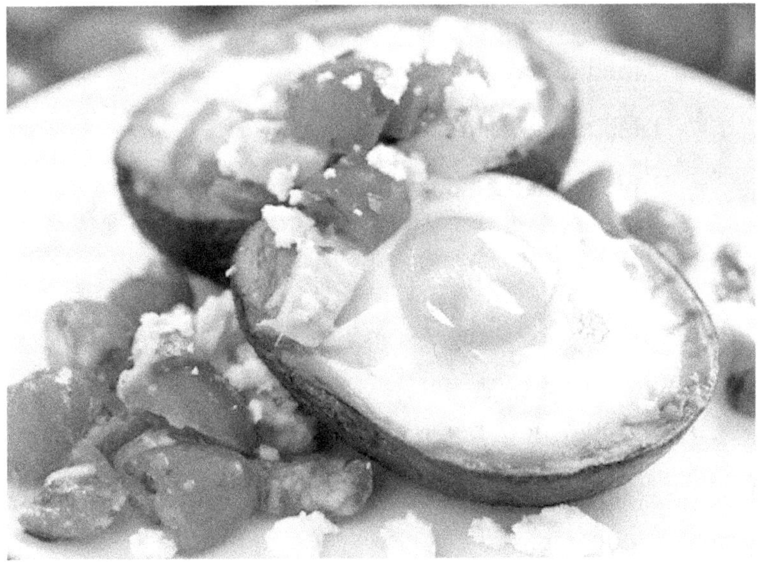

Do you love those quick breakfast recipes that you can prepare in less than 30 minutes? This one will really amaze you with the flavors. No one will believe that you can prepare a gourmet breakfast for you and your family in only 20 minutes. The avocado will provide healthy fats that will keep you full. The process of preparation is so easy, so everyone can do it. Double the **Ingredients** to feed your whole family. Let's start preparing this awesome breakfast!

Servings:2

Cooking time: 20 minutes

Ingredients

- 2 large eggs
- 1 medium avocado
- 1 tablespoon shredded cheese
- 1 piece bacon, cooked and crumbled
- Salt to taste

Instructions

1. Cut your avocado in half. Take the pit out. With a spoon, remove some of the middle. This way, you will have enough space for one egg.

2. Place the filled avocado on a muffin tin. This will keep them in place.

3. Crack the egg. Add it in the pitted avocado. Repeat with the second egg.

4. Sprinkle with salt. Add cheese and top with bacon.

5. Preheat oven to 425 degrees. Baking time varies from 14 to 16 minutes. Enjoy!

Cream cheese pancakes

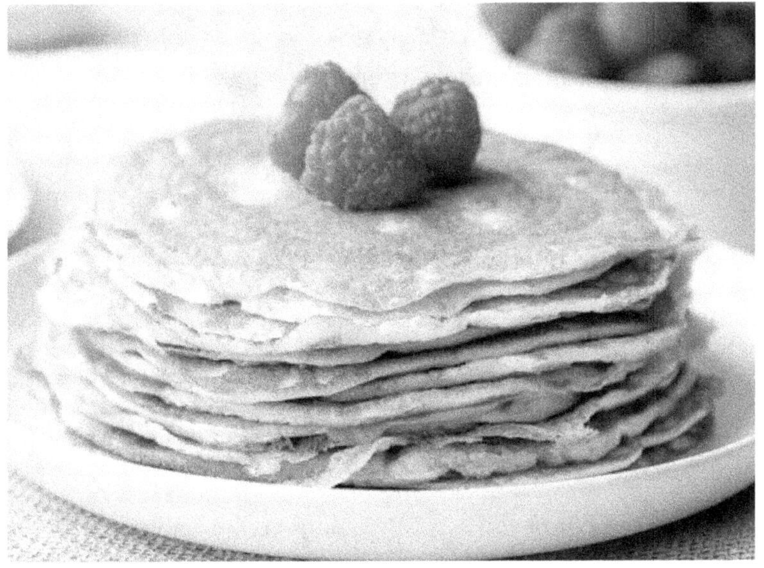

Who doesn't love a fresh batch of pancakes in the morning? Even if you are not consuming any carbs, you can still enjoy the fluffiness of the pancakes. This recipe will guide you in the process of making the best ones. The cream cheese will add a versatile taste, while the eggs will make the pancakes so fluffy. In a short time, it will become your favorite for sure. So, let's get started!

Servings:4

Cooking time: 12 minutes

Ingredients

- 2 large eggs
- 2oz cream cheese, softened
- 1 teaspoon granulated sugar substitute
- 1/2 teaspoon cinnamon

Instructions

1. To make it easier, mix everything in a blender or food processor. This will save you so much time and effort.

2. Leave the batter to rest. In 2 minutes, the bubbles will all settle down.

3. Heat some oil in a frying pan. Add ¼ of the batter. Fry the pancake for 2 minutes, flip, and cook for one more minute. Repeat until you finish the batter.

Savory muffins with sausage

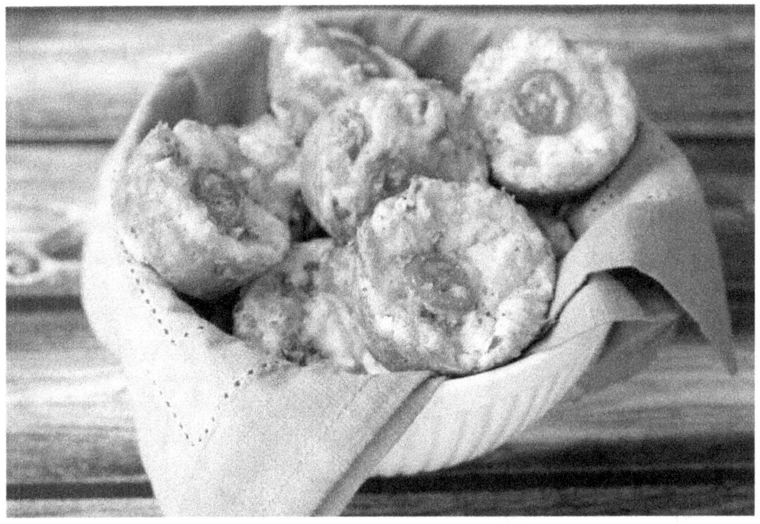

Are you looking for the perfect breakfast on the go? Muffins are your top choice. They are easy to transport and prepare ahead, so this will become your favorite recipe. In a total of 20 minutes, you will have a whole batch of muffins ready. This is the kind of breakfast that will feed the entire family.

Servings: 12

Cooking time: 20 minutes

Ingredients

- 1/2 cup shredded Cheese

- 1/2 Pound Ground Sausage, cooked

- 10 Eggs

- 1/3 Cup Cream Cheese, softened at room temperature

- 1/2 cup finely chopped red bell pepper

- 1/2 Cup Chopped Green Onions

- Salt

- Pepper

Instructions

1. Start by greasing your muffin tin. Preheat oven to 400 degrees too.

2. Remove the excess fat off the cooked sausage meat.

3. With a hand mixer, beat together the eggs and softened cream cheese. You should come to a smooth mixture.

4. Add in the chopped vegetables. Mix well.

5. Fill the muffin tin. Leave some space, because the muffins will rise. Fill about ½ or ⅔ of each. Bake for 10 minutes and enjoy!

Avocado and patty sandwich

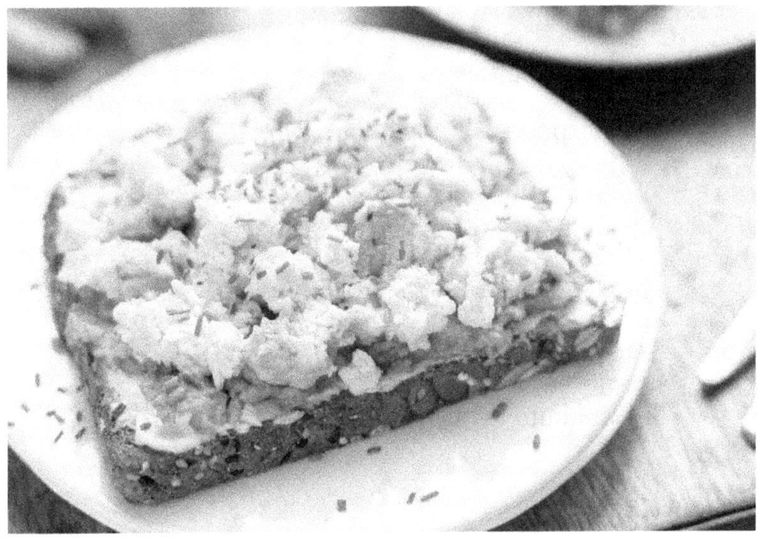

Sandwiches are the perfect food that is easy to transport. Whether it is a picnic, a lunch for work or merely a prep-ahead breakfast, this recipe will prove to be so helpful for you. It is different from any traditional recipe because it doesn't have any bread. It is replaced with a patty so that you will feel full without consuming any carbs. So, let's start with the preparations!

Servings: 1

Cooking time: 20 minutes

Ingredients

- 1 large egg
- 2 sausage patties
- 2 tablespoons shredded cheddar
- 1 tablespoon cream cheese, softened at room temperature
- Salt, pepper to taste
- 1/4–1/2 teaspoon sriracha
- 1/4 medium avocado, sliced

Instructions

1. Heat oil in a skillet. Cook the patties according to the **Instructions** given on the package. Remove and set aside.

2. In a bowl, add the cream cheese. Add the cheddar and mix. Pop it in the micro for about 20-30 seconds, or until melted. Remove, add sriracha, mix, and set aside.

3. Crack the egg and fry it. Season your omelet to taste.

4. Assemble your sandwich. The patties will be the buns: layer egg, cheese, and chopped avocado. Enjoy while still warm, or preserve for later.

No carb pizza recipe

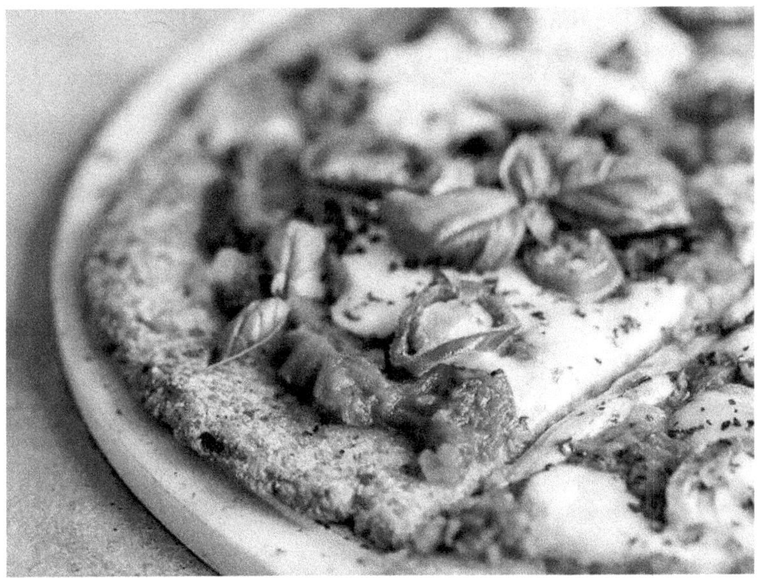

It is not a secret that pizza is everyone's guilty pleasure. With this recipe in your hands, you will be able to enjoy the decadent taste without consuming carbs. It is packed with the most delicate flavors and made to satisfy your tastebuds. Everyone will be amazed by this recipe, that doesn't stand out from the original one. So, head to the kitchen and start with the preparations!

Servings:8

Cooking time: 40 minutes

Ingredients

- 1/2 cup heavy cream
- 12 eggs
- 8 oz sausage
- 1/2 teaspoon salt
- 1/4 teaspoon pepper
- 1 cup shredded cheese
- 2 cups peppers, chopped

Instructions

1. Cook the peppers in the micro for about 3 minutes. Remove and set aside.

2. Cook the sausage in a skillet over medium heat. Remove and set aside.

3. In a bowl, mix the eggs and cream. Season with salt and pepper.

4. Add the mixture from the bowl into the skillet. Cook for 5 minutes.

5. Put it in a preheated oven to 350 degrees. Bake for 15 minutes.

6. Remove and add the sausage, cheese, and peppers.

7. Return to the oven and broil for three more minutes.

8. Let it set down for 5 minutes before you cut a piece.
Enjoy!

Breakfast bagels

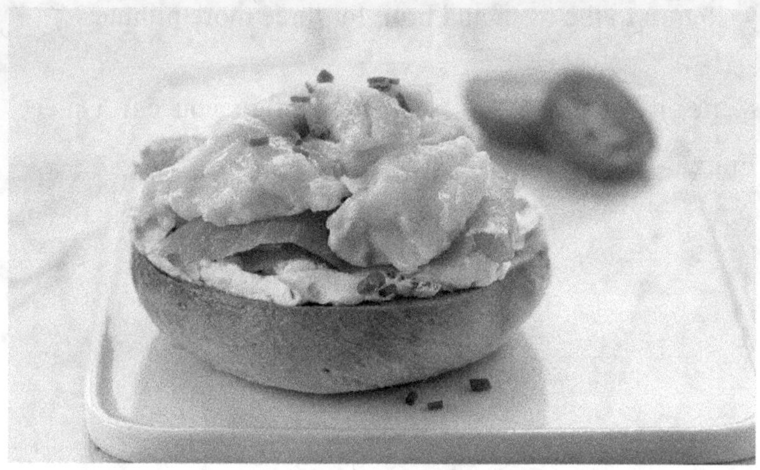

Do you love fresh bagels for breakfast? This recipe will soon become your favorite. You will be able to make your favorite bagel sandwiches and enjoy them in the mornings. The simple method won't take you long, which is very convenient for busy people. It won't take you lot of time, so let's get started!

Servings:6

Cooking time: 20 minutes

Ingredients

- 1 cup shredded mozzarella
- 2 large eggs
- 1/2 cup grated parmesan
- 2 tablespoons bagel seasoning

Instructions

1. Preheat oven to 375.

2. In a bowl, add shredded mozzarella and parmesan. Mix in the eggs.

3. When it is well combined, divide the mixture into six equal parts. Place them in a greased donut shape pan.

4. Sprinkle with the seasoning on top. Bake for about seventeen minutes or until the cheese melts and gets a slight brown color on top.

Lunch Recipes

Beef lettuce wraps

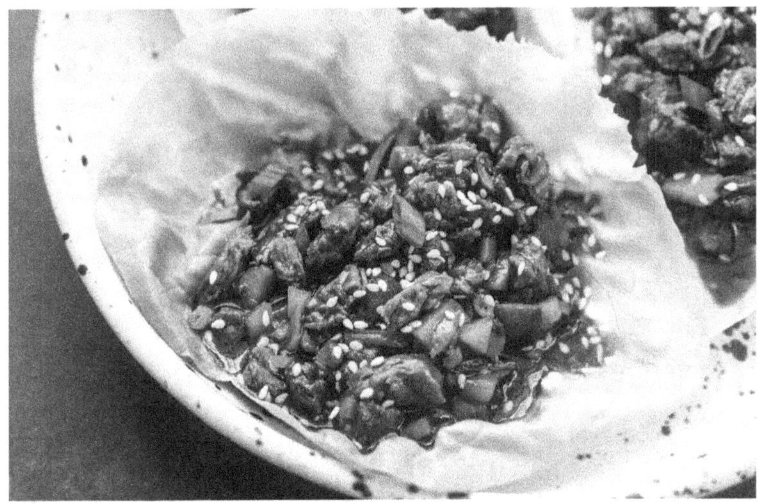

Are you looking for a delicious gourmet lunch? This recipe will show you how to do it in less than 30 minutes. The aromatic sauces will bring a modern twist to the meat. The lettuce will help you create wraps, that you can enjoy without any guilt.

Servings: 4

Cooking time: 25 minutes

Ingredients

- 1 lb. ground beef
- 2 teaspoons oil

- 1-2 heads iceberg lettuce
- 1 T fish sauce (see notes)
- 2 tablespoons water
- 1 tablespoon Sriracha Sauce
- 1/2 cup thinly sliced green onion
- zest from one large lime
- 1 1/2 tablespoon lime juice

Instructions

1. Heat oil in a pan over medium-high. Cook the beef until brown, while breaking it down.

2. Mix fish sauce, Sriracha, and water in a small bowl.

3. Wash the lettuce and cut it into quarters to make the cups.

4. Add sauce mixture in the pan. Stir and let it sizzle. Cook until the water has evaporated.

5. Turn off the heat. Add lime zest, lime juice, sliced green onions. Mix well.

6. Fill the lettuce cups with the meat mixture. Enjoy!

Cucumber Tuna rolls

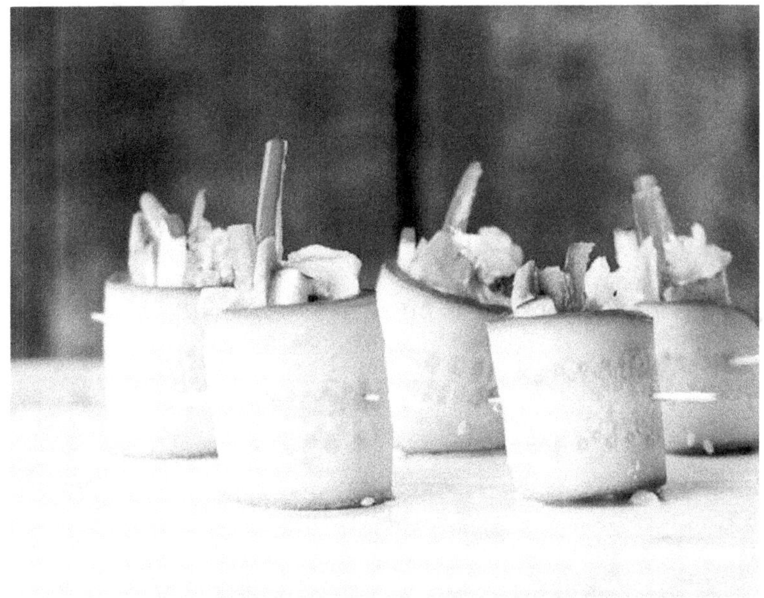

Are you looking for the perfect 5-minute lunch that you can easily make? This recipe will show you how to make delicious tuna rolls. They are made of cucumber, so you don't have to worry about your carb intake.

Servings:

Cooking time: 5 minutes

Ingredients

- 1 can of tuna
- 1 medium cucumber
- 2 teaspoons sriracha
- 1 tablespoon mayo (for tuna mixture)
- Avocado, sliced
- 2 teaspoons garlic powder
- Salt
- Pepper

Sauce:

- 2 tablespoon mayo
- 2 tsp sriracha

Instructions

1. With the help of a vegetable peeler, slice the cucumbers into thin strips.

2. Drain the tuna can and add in sriracha, garlic powder, salt, and pepper. Mix well until combined. The mixture shouldn't be too wet.

3. Place the strips on a flat surface. Spread the tuna. Place avocado slice and roll the cucumber strips.

4. To make the sauce, simply mix mayo and sriracha. Drizzle on top and enjoy!

No carb empanadas

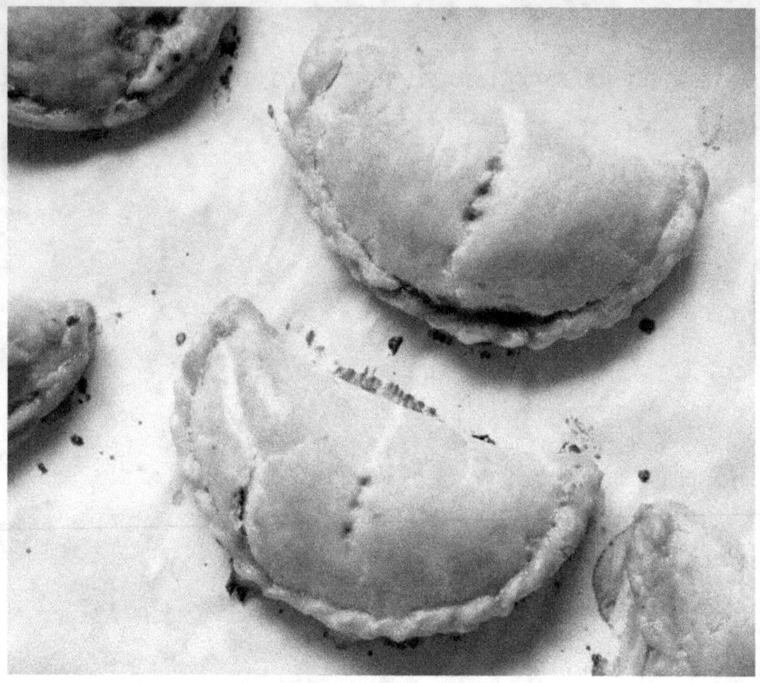

Are you looking for the ultimate no carb recipe for empanadas? This one will really surprise you with the flavors. The combination of chicken and different types of cheese will tickle your tastebuds. This meal will soon become your favorite, so let's get started!

Servings:4

Cooking time:35 minutes

Ingredients

- 3 oz cream cheese
- 1½ cups shredded mozzarella
- 1 egg, whisked
- 1¼ cup almond flour

Filling:

- 2 cups cooked and shredded chicken
- ⅓ cup hot sauce

Instructions

1. Preheating the oven to 425 degrees.

2. Put the mozzarella and cheese in a bowl. Pop them in the microwave until melted. Stop to mix, then return again.

3. Add almond flour and the whisked egg. Mix well until you make a nice dough. If it sticks to your fingers, add some more flour.

4. Roll it with plastic wrap on top. Once it is flat and thin, cut out circle shapes.

5. Lay them on a greased cooking pan.

6. Mix the shredded chicken with the sauce. Add one spoon into half of the circles. Fold and close each one.

7. Bake your empanadas for 12 minutes. Enjoy!

Zucchini casserole

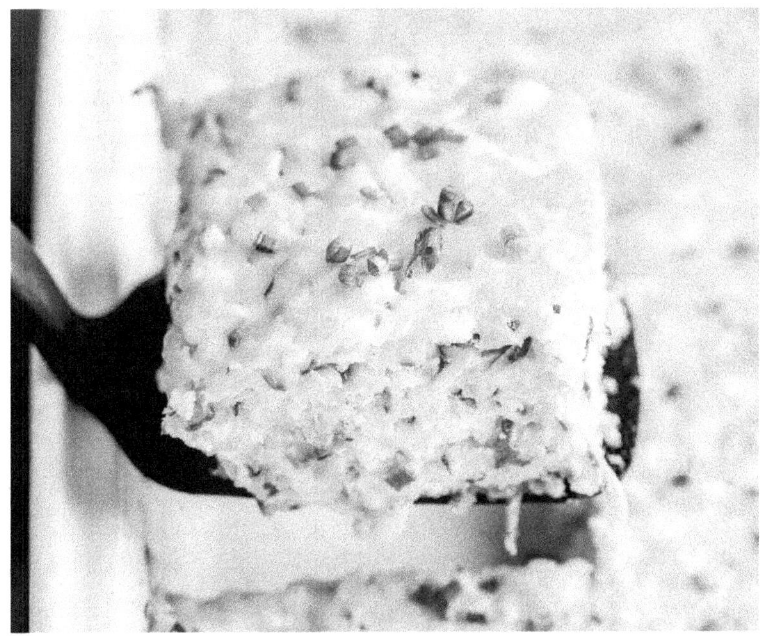

Do you want an easy recipe for lunch? This one is prepared in less than 5 minutes. You just need to put a few **Ingredients** in the blender and it will do the mixing for you. Pour everything in your casserole dish, bake, and your gourmet lunch is ready!

Servings:6

Cooking time:35 minutes

Ingredients

- 8 egg whites
- 2 cups shredded zucchini, drained
- 3 wedges light swiss cheese
- 1/2 cup cottage cheese
- 3 tablespoons bacon crumbles
- 1/4 cup unsweetened almond milk
- Salt

Instructions

1. Preheat the oven to 350 degrees.

2. Grease your casserole dish with cooking spray.

3. Put the shredded zucchini.

4. Place the other **Ingredients** in a blender. Pulse until combined. Pour it over the zucchini in the dish.

5. Bake for about 30 minutes, or until golden brown. Enjoy!

Stuffed jalapeno peppers

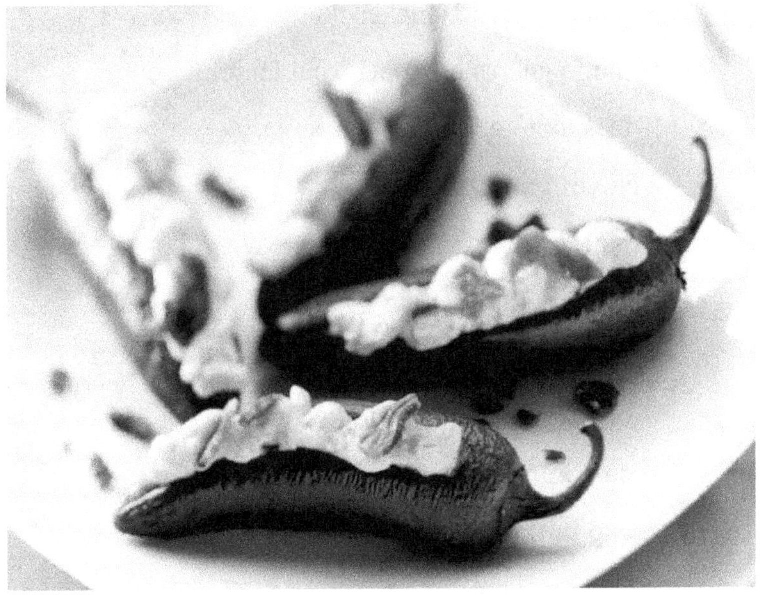

If you are tired of having the usual chicken for lunch, then check this awesome recipe. With being so delicious and spicy, this stuffed jalapeno recipe will become your personal favorite. Serve it with creamy and tasty ranch dressing for the full enjoyment.

Servings:5

Cooking time: 35 minutes

Ingredients

- 8 ounces ground chicken
- 10 large jalapeño peppers, cut lengthwise
- ½ teaspoon onion powder
- 2 cloves garlic, minced
- 4 ounces cream cheese, softened
- ½ teaspoon salt
- 4 strips bacon, cooked and crumbled
- ¼ cup shredded mozzarella cheese
- ½ cup crumbled blue cheese, divided
- ¼ cup buffalo wing sauce
- Ranch dressing, for serving

Instructions

1. Preheat the oven to 350 degrees.

2. Line the baking sheet with paper. Remove the seeds from the peppers and place them on the paper.

3. Heat a skillet over medium heat. Add chicken, garlic, onion powder, and salt. Cook until the chicken is completely cooked. Remove and add to a big bowl.

4. In the same bowl, add in the three types of cheese (leave out ¼ cup of blue cheese crumbles aside) and the sauce. Mix well.

5. Fill each pepper with this mixture. Top with the rest of the blue cheese and bacon.

6. Bake the peppers for 30 minutes, or until golden brown. Enjoy!

Cheeseburger casserole

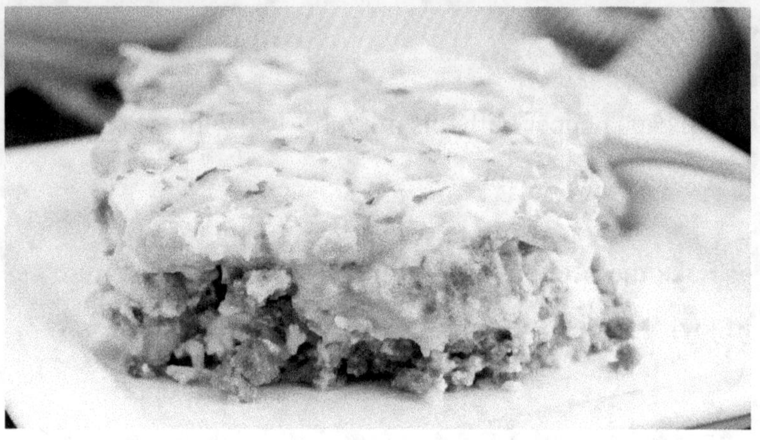

A casserole is the simplest dish that everyone can make. All you need to do is layer a few carefully picked **Ingredients**. This recipe shows you a very delicious combination of flavors. They are meant to amaze every foodie out there, eager to try some delicious foods that don't have carbs.

Servings:6

Cooking time: 45 minutes

Ingredients

- 2 cup cauliflower, chopped
- 1 lb ground meat
- 1/4 cup cheddar cheese, shredded

- 2 teaspoon steak seasoning

- 1/2 cup cheddar cheese, shredded

- 4 oz cream cheese cut into cubes

- 1 tablespoon butter, melted

- 1/2 cup heavy cream

- 2 eggs

Instructions

1. Preheat oven to 400 degrees.

2. Cook the cauliflower in micro five minutes.

3. In a pan, heat some oil. Cook the ground beef until brown. Add steak seasoning for a better taste.

4. Add the cooked cauliflower in the skillet. Add cream cheese and only 1/4 cup of cheddar cheese. Mix well until combined.

5. Pour the mixture into a casserole dish of your choice.

6. In a separate bowl, whisk the eggs with cream and butter. Pour this mixture in the casserole dish. Top with the rest of the cheese.

7. Bake for 30 minutes.

Zoodles with parmesan

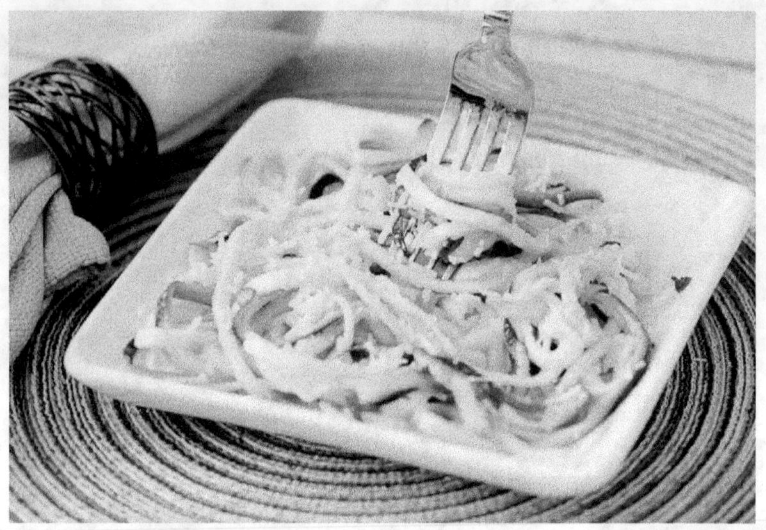

Pasta is one of the things that you will miss the most. But, not with this recipe. It will show you how to prepare the perfect creamy zoodles that will replace the carb-rich paste recipes. It is easy to be prepared, so you can enjoy the rest of the time.

Servings: 2

Cooking time: 10 minutes

Ingredients

- 4-5 medium zucchini, spiralized

- 1 tablespoon butter

- ¼ cup Parmesan cheese

- 4 oz cream cheese

- 3 tablespoons milk

- salt

- Pepper

- 2 cloves garlic, minced

- sliced cherry tomatoes

Instructions

1. Place the butter in a large pan. Set to medium low heat. Add garlic and cook for a minute.

2. Add the cream cheese and milk. Cook until everything melts and you end up with a sauce.

3. Add the zoodles. Mix them well, so that they will get evenly covered with the sauce.

4. Add parmesan and continue to cook. It is finished when the zoodles are softened. Garnish with cherry tomatoes on the plate. Enjoy!

Desserts

Chocolate frosty recipe

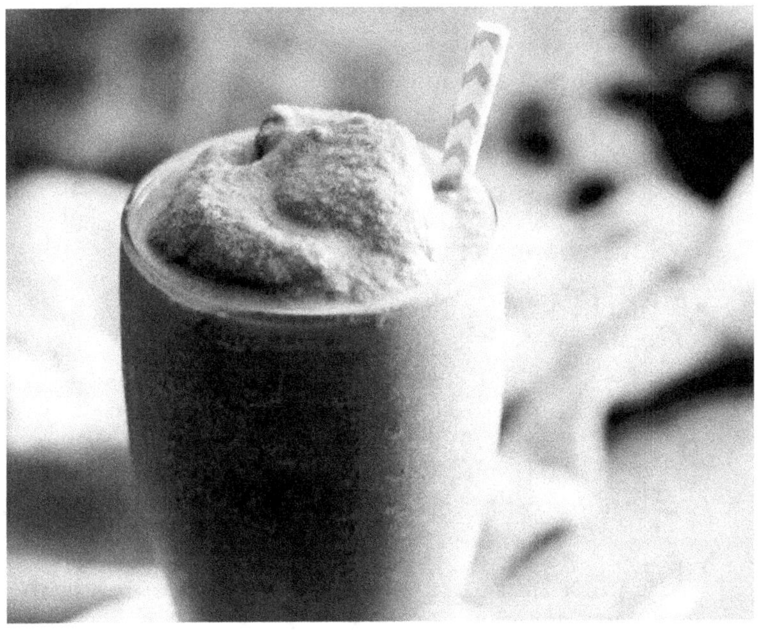

Can't control your chocolate cravings? This is the recipe that will change that. The chocolate frosty is prepared in only 5 minutes. You will end up with one decadent and creamy dessert that will blow your mind. Finally, here is a dessert that won't make you gain weight!

Servings:2

Cooking time: 35 minutes

Ingredients

- 2 tablespoons unsweetened cocoa powder
- 1 cup heavy whipping cream
- 5 drops liquid stevia, or other carb-free sweeteners of your choice
- 1 teaspoon vanilla extract
- 1 tablespoon almond butter

Instructions

Add the heavy cream in a bowl. Beat using a hand mixer.

Add the other **Ingredients**. Blend until you reach the consistency of thick whipping cream.

Pop it in the freezer for about 30 minutes. Serve and enjoy!

Chocolate brownies

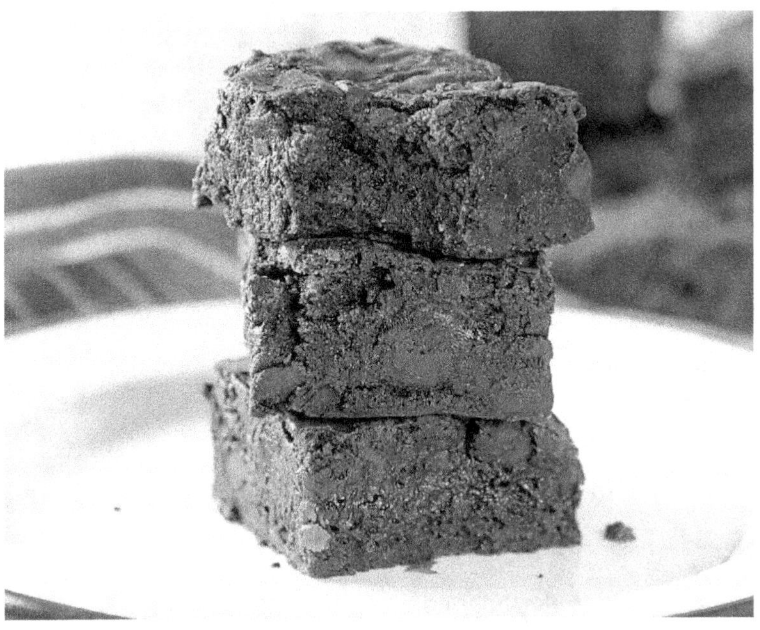

Do you miss the taste of the chewy and chocolatey brownies, ready to melt in your mouth? This recipe won't disappoint you. It will give you the complete **Instructions** on how to make the best brownies that don't have any carbs at all. Everything that you need to do is follow this easy recipe!

Servings: 16

Cooking time: 30 minutes

Ingredients

- 1 cup almond butter,
- 1/2 cup unsweetened cocoa powder
- 2/3 cup powdered erythritol
- 1 tablespoon coconut flour
- 2 tablespoons peanut butter powder, sugar-free
- 1 tablespoon butter, melted
- 3 large eggs, room temperature
- 1/2 teaspoon of baking powder
- 2 tablespoons water
- 1 ½ teaspoon pure vanilla extract
- 1/2 cup dark chocolate chips, sugar-free
- 1/4 teaspoons salt

Instructions

1. Preheat the oven to 325 degrees.

2. Grease your baking pan.

3. In a large bowl, add all of the listed **Ingredients**. With a hand mixer, mix everything well together until thoroughly combined. When done, add in the chocolate chips.

4. Pour the mixture in the pan. Bake for twenty minutes, or until the edges are set. Don't overbake because the center should be chewy. Let it set before you cut the pieces.

No bake orange creamsicles

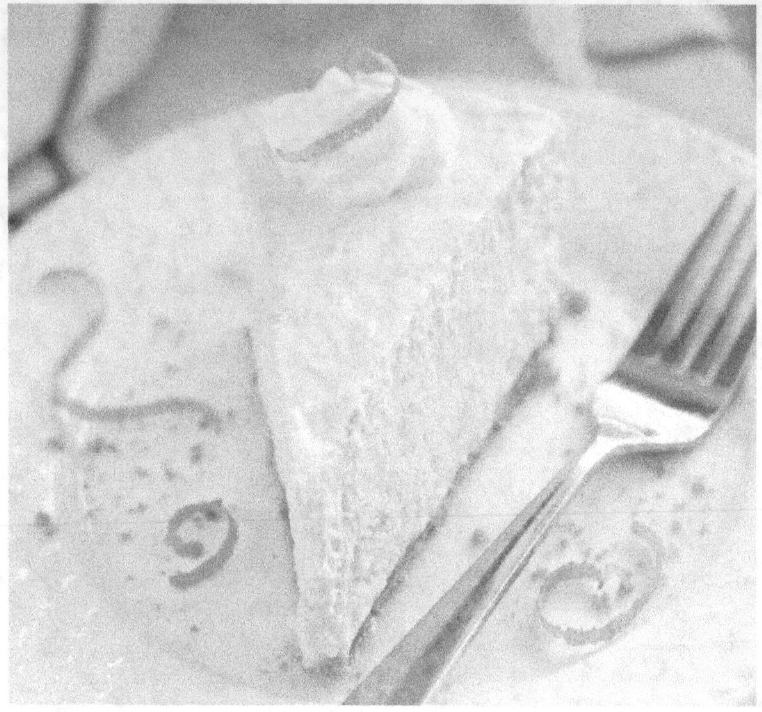

A creamy and decadent dessert is a must for every day. This recipe will show you how to prepare delicious creamsicles without much effort. Everything that you need to do is mix four **Ingredients** and put them in the freezer. Your dessert will wait for you!

Servings:8

Cooking time: 3 hours 15 minutes

Ingredients

- ½ cup Water
- 1 cup Heavy Cream
- Orange Zest
- 1 30-ounce package Sugar-Free Orange Jello

Instructions

1. In a pot, boil the water. Add in the jello. Mix until it dissolves completely.

2. Sprinkle some orange zest. Add in the heavy cream and mix everything.

3. Pour in small silicone molds of your choice.

4. Place in the freezer for 3 hours.

Creamy raspberry balls

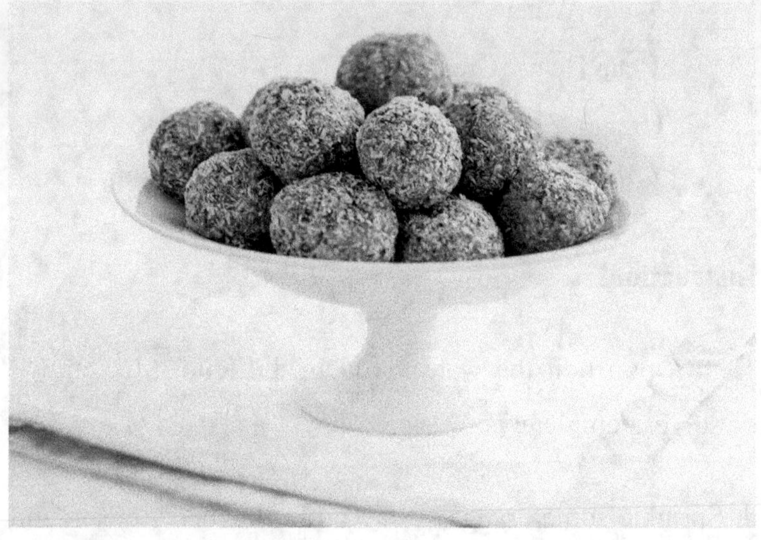

Do you like desserts with fruity flavors? Here is another easy recipe for you. Raspberries are very delicious and will give a rich flavor to any dessert when added. They are flavorful, fresh, and extremely creamy, so make sure that you don't miss this recipe!

Servings:8

Cooking time:1 hr 30 minutes

Ingredients

- 3.50 oz raspberries

- 2 tablespoons softened butter

- 2 tablespoon finely ground almond flour

- 1 teaspoon freshly squeezed lemon juice

- 2 tablespoon granulated erythritol

Instructions

1. Heat the fruit in a pot on low to medium heat. Simmer for 10-15 minutes, or until the liquid is dissolved. Stir occasionally, until you reach a dark paste.

2. Add the raspberry paste in a large bowl. Add in the other **Ingredients**. Mix well until fully combined.

3. Let it chill in the freezer for ten to fifteen minutes. Remove and shape the balls. Chill them for one more hour. Enjoy!

Mango cheesecake balls

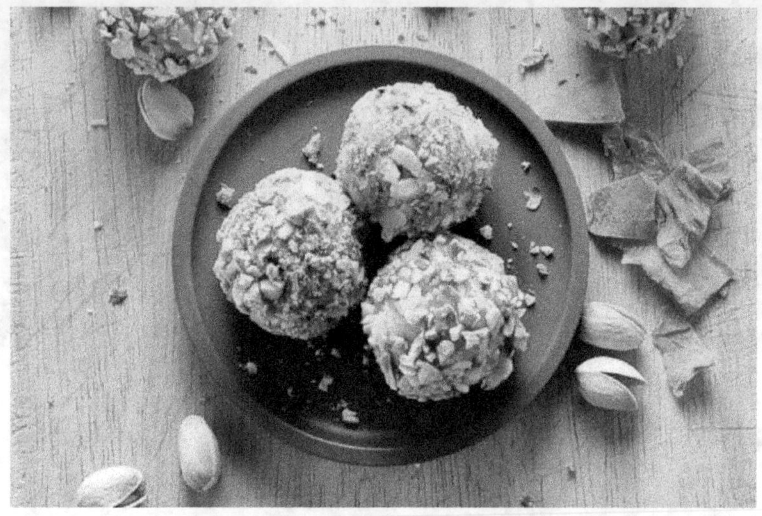

Ready for another spectacular dessert? These cheesecake balls are enhanced by the awesome taste of the mango. The best thing is that you can shape them into whatever form you like. This is the kind of aromatic and decadent dessert that you wished. It won't take you much of your precious time, so get to work now!

Servings:6

Cooking time: 2 hours

Ingredients

- 75 grams Fresh Mango, diced
- ¼ cup Butter, softened
- 6 oz Cream Cheese, softened
- ¼ cup Walnuts, roughly chopped
- 1 tbsp Vanilla
- 1 tsp Ground Cinnamon
- 2 packets stevia

Instructions

1. Blend the mango until you reach a thick puree.

2. Add cheese, butter, cinnamon, vanilla, and stevia. Blend again until you reach a smooth mixture.

3. Add walnuts into the silicone molds. Fill with the mixture.

4. Freezing time is somewhere between one and two hours. Enjoy!

Chocolate glazed donuts

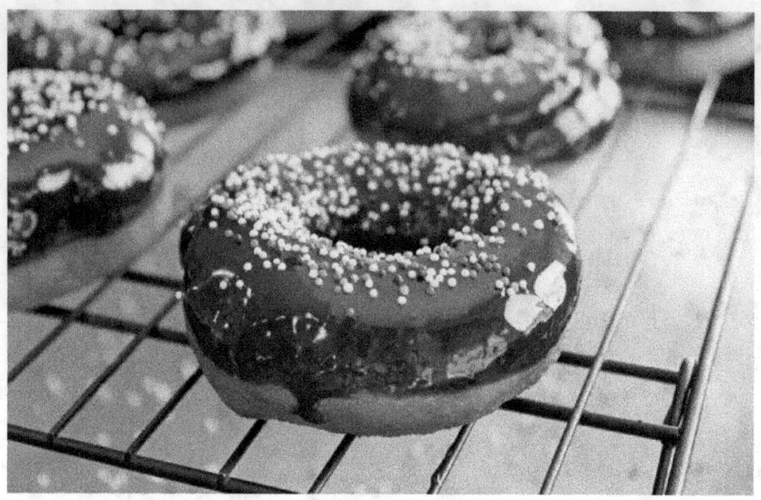

Can you make donuts without flour? The answer is yes. But there is more. You can make the tastiest donuts without relying on carbs. And this recipe will show you how to do it. In a short time, you will get addicted to these decadent chocolate-covered donuts. So, check the easy method and start now!

Servings:9

Cooking time:20 minutes

Ingredients

- 2 eggs

- ¼ cup cream cheese

- 1 ½ cup almond flour

- ⅓ cup butter, softened

- 1 teaspoon baking powder

- 6 teaspoons keto sweetener

- ½ cup sugar-free chocolate

Instructions

1. Preheat oven to 350 degrees. Grease your mold.

2. In a bowl, mix the butter, cream cheese, and eggs. Beat with a mixer until smooth.

3. In a second bowl, mix all of the dry **Ingredients**: almond flour, baking powder, and sweetener.

4. Add the dry **Ingredients** into the other mixture. Beat well.

5. Pour the mixture into the molds, leaving some space so that they can rise. Bake for about 20-25 minutes. Set them aside to cool.

6. Prepare the glaze by simply melting the chocolate. Dip the donuts and let them harden.

Peanut butter popsicles

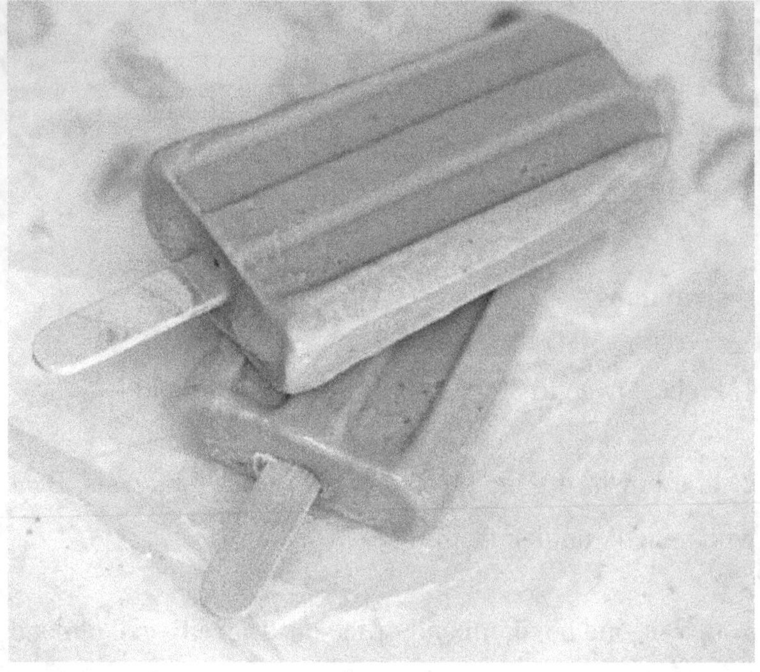

The list of recipes isn't complete without these delicious popsicles. The peanut butter adds an exquisite flavor, while the chocolate completes the recipe. You can make them in only 10 minutes so that you won't lose any of your precious time. Let's get started!

Servings:6

Cooking time: 10 minutes

Ingredients

- 2 tablespoons peanut butter
- ½ cup coconut cream
- 1 cup almond milk
- 2 tablespoons stevia

½ cup unsweetened chocolate chips, melted

Instructions

1. Add all of the **Ingredients** in a blender, except for the chocolate chips. Blend until well combined.

2. Grease your silicone mold with a little bit of spray. Add the mixture into the molds. Add a wooden stick at the end.

3. Put them in the freezer for 3 hours.

4. Once they are completely firm, drizzle with melted chocolate.

Conclusion

Once you have come to the end of this cookbook, you will know how to prepare the tastiest no carb dishes. The recipes can be made on an everyday basis, so they are easy to implement in your current lifestyle. We have shared the secrets to preparing the best desserts that taste as good as the traditional ones. Also, you found a wide range of recipes that you can make for lunch and dinner. And let's not forget about the breakfast ideas that are meant to make your life easier.

Each and every recipe in this cookbook has goals: to help you lose weight and save you cooking time. Your strong will and motivation together with our useful tips will pave your way to success

We wish you happy cooking!.

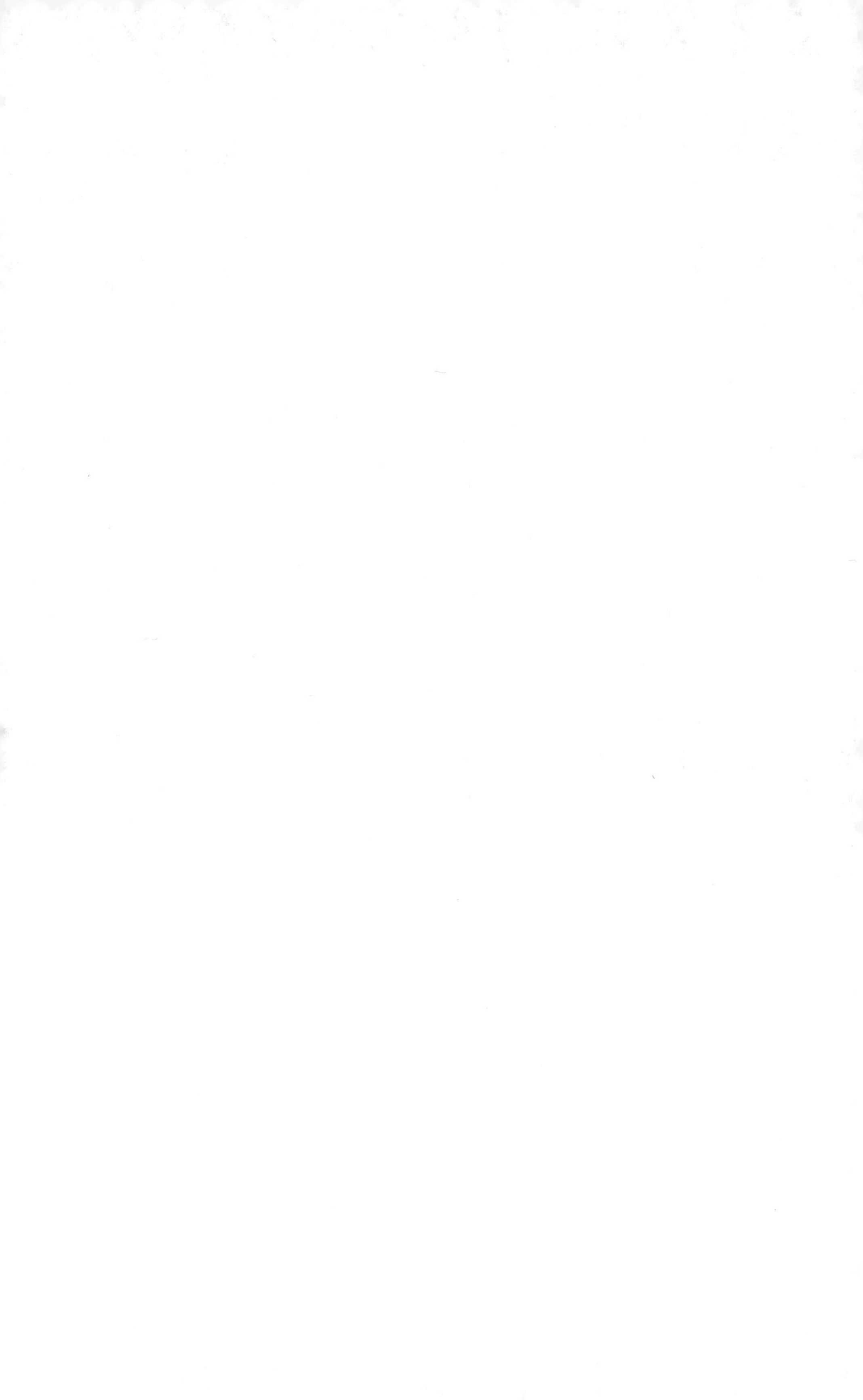